Respiratory Syncytial Virus

**Understanding, Managing, and Preventing RSV
Across Ages, Amidst Pandemics, and Towards a
Healthier Future**

Olivia Winterbourne, MPH

Table of Contents

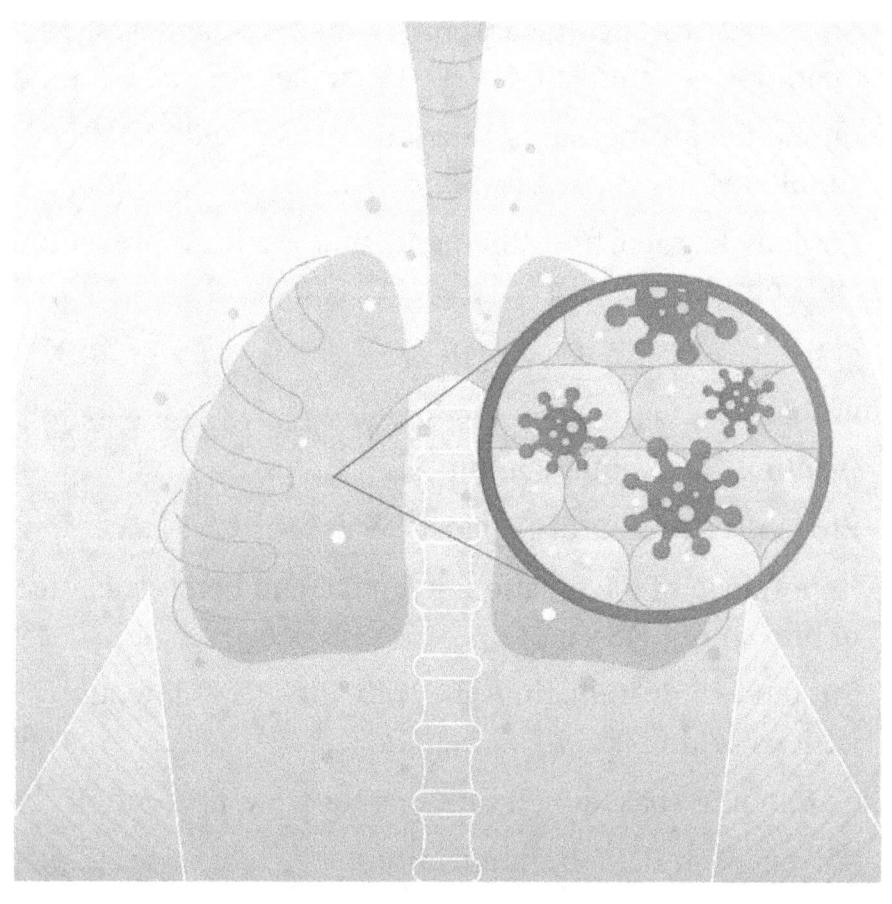

Introduction

In a world marked by the unseen, where the invisible threads of a virus weave through our lives, there exists a silent adversary that traverses generations, challenging our respiratory health and resilience – Respiratory Syncytial Virus (RSV). It impact across ages, unsettling the very breath that sustains us, especially amidst the turbulent waves of pandemics. Yet, within this landscape of uncertainty, knowledge becomes our beacon, our shield against the unknown.

Welcome to *"Respiratory Syncytial Virus: Understanding, Managing, and Preventing RSV Across Ages, Amidst Pandemics, and Towards a Healthier Future."* As an expert in the realm of health, my journey through the intricacies of RSV has led me to unveil the multifaceted layers of this viral entity that hides within the air we breathe.

This book isn't merely about a virus; it's a quest for comprehension, a revelation of resilience, and a guidepost towards a healthier tomorrow. Its relevance transcends the confines of a medical journal; it's a testament to the interconnectedness of our lives, the vulnerabilities that traverse age brackets, and the relentless pursuit of safeguarding our well-being.

As we embark on this journey together, I invite you to join me in exploring the landscape of RSV – from its origins, the historical footprints that led us to its discovery, to the nuanced intricacies of its impact on infants, children, adults, and vulnerable populations. Together, we shall navigate through the labyrinth of symptoms, delve into diagnostic procedures, explore available treatments, and unearth the significance of preventive measures.

However, this book isn't just a compendium of facts and figures; it's a roadmap toward empowerment, resilience, and hope. Along the way, you'll uncover the latest advancements in RSV vaccines, promising glimpses of a future where we stand equipped against this silent assailant.

As I guide you through the chapters meticulously crafted within these pages, I promise you an odyssey filled with enlightenment, a tapestry woven with empathy, and a beacon of trust backed by rigorous research and expertise. Yet, I won't reveal all within these introductory lines; there are tales untold, revelations yet to be unveiled, and discoveries awaiting your eager curiosity.

Fear not, dear reader, for within these pages, we shall tackle every doubt, dispel every fear, and emerge armed with knowledge and understanding. So, I invite you to embark on this journey with an open mind, a thirst for knowledge, and a resolve to conquer the mysteries of Respiratory Syncytial Virus. Together, we shall stride towards a future where breath is no longer held captive, but a symbol of resilience and health.

Are you ready to uncover the secrets of RSV, traverse through pandemics, and pave a path towards a healthier future? If so, let us embark on this transformative odyssey together.

Chapter 1

Understanding Respiratory Syncytial Virus

Respiratory Syncytial Virus (RSV) is a usual kind of germ that causes problems in our breathing. It mostly goes into our lungs and the paths we use to breathe. This virus is pretty easy to spread because it moves around very quickly. When someone who has RSV coughs or sneezes, tiny drops from their mouth can carry the virus and go into the air. If these drops get into someone else's mouth or nose, they might get infected too. Also, if you touch something that has the virus on it, like a toy or a doorknob, and then touch your face, the virus can get into your body that way."

RSV is like a tiny invisible thing that can make us sick if we're not careful. So, it's important to try to stay away from people who are sick with RSV, wash our hands often, and avoid touching our face too much. These are some of the ways to help stop the virus from spreading and making more people sick.

Brief history and discovery of RSV

RSV's story began a long time ago, in the 1950s. Scientists were studying sick chimpanzees, and they found a tiny thing they called 'chimpanzee coryza agent' (CCA), which was making these chimps ill. Later on, in 1957, a smart scientist named Robert M. Chanock noticed something important. He realized that the same tiny thing that made the chimpanzees sick was also making children sick with breathing problems.

More research showed that this tiny thing was quite common in babies and young kids. They found out that many children got sick from this 'thing' when they were very young. Scientists then decided to give it a new name, 'human orthopneumovirus,' but most people know it as human respiratory syncytial virus or hRSV for short.

So, this virus has been around for quite a while, and scientists have been learning more and more about it over the years. They found out it's a common bug that can cause breathing troubles, especially in little ones.

Over time, more and more scientists joined in to study RSV. They wanted to understand how it made children sick and why it was so good at spreading. Even though scientists discovered RSV many years ago, the story doesn't end there. They're still working hard, trying to find better ways to protect kids and everyone else from this tricky little bug.

So, the history of RSV is like a big puzzle that scientists have been solving for decades. Each discovery they make helps us understand this virus better and find new ways to keep everyone healthy.

Importance of RSV as a respiratory illness

RSV is a pretty big deal when it comes to breathing sickness. It's a germ that can make babies, little kids, older adults, and folks with weaker immune systems really sick. Imagine it as a common troublemaker causing problems in people's breathing tubes and lungs."

It's especially tough on babies – the ones younger than one year old. RSV is so sneaky that it often causes a condition called bronchiolitis, where the tiny airways in their lungs get all swollen and it's hard for them to breathe. In fact, in the United States, RSV is the main reason behind bronchiolitis and pneumonia in babies under one year old."

But RSV doesn't just pick on babies. It can also hit older adults hard, especially those over 65 years old. And if someone already has problems with their lungs or heart, RSV can make things even worse for them. It's like this germ has a knack for making breathing really difficult for some folks."

So, you see, RSV is a big deal because it can cause serious breathing problems for different people, from tiny babies to older adults. That's why doctors and scientists keep an eye on it and work hard to find ways to protect everyone from getting really sick.

Impact of RSV on vulnerable populations.

RSV is like a troublemaker for certain groups of people who are more sensitive or fragile when it comes to sickness. These are the folks who need extra care because they might get really sick from this virus. We're talking about tiny babies born too early or those who are very young, kids with special health problems like lung or heart issues, and older adults who are 65 years or older.

Usually, when a healthy person catches RSV, they might feel a bit sick for about a week, but then they start feeling better. It's like having a cold that goes away after a while. But for these vulnerable folks, RSV is like a big fight for their health. It can make them seriously sick, and sometimes it can even be life-threatening.

For babies, especially those who are born early, RSV can make it hard for them to breathe properly. Imagine trying to eat when you're having a tough time catching your breath – it's really difficult! That's what happens to these little ones fighting against RSV. It's not just about feeling sick; it affects their eating and can make them very uncomfortable.

Even after the RSV infection goes away, it can leave behind some problems. For example, it might make these vulnerable individuals more likely to have other breathing troubles later on. RSV can bring along friends like pneumonia, which is a really serious lung infection. It can also increase the chances of getting conditions like asthma or COPD, which make it hard to breathe in the long run.

So, for these special groups of people, RSV isn't just a small bug that makes them feel a bit under the weather. It's a big deal that can seriously affect their health, making it hard for them to breathe properly and sometimes causing lasting problems. That's why doctors and families of these vulnerable folks work extra hard to protect them from getting sick with RSV.

In essence, RSV poses a substantial threat to vulnerable populations such as premature babies, infants with health issues, and older adults, causing more severe symptoms, interfering with their breathing and eating, and potentially leading to long-term health complications. This expanded explanation aims to simplify the impact of RSV on these groups, highlighting the challenges they face and the importance of safeguarding their health against this virus.

Current state of RSV research

The Centers for Disease Control and Prevention (CDC) is actively conducting and supporting basic research on RSV to improve our understanding of the virus and how it causes disease, as well as factors in animals and humans that affect susceptibility to RSV infection.

The CDC is like a team of health detectives who work really hard to understand how viruses like RSV make us sick and find ways to keep us healthy. They're doing lots of important research to learn more about RSV and how it causes problems in our bodies. They want to know why some people get sicker from RSV than others and what things might make us more likely to catch this virus."

One important thing they're studying is how RSV affects both animals and humans. This helps them understand why some animals or people might get RSV more easily than others. By learning this, they can try to find better ways to protect us from getting sick with RSV.

The CDC is also focused on keeping an eye on when and how RSV spreads during different times of the year. They have special systems – like the National Respiratory and Enteric Virus Surveillance System (NREVSS) and the National Syndromic Surveillance Program (NSSP) – that help them keep track of how many people are getting sick from RSV. These systems help them know about the trends of RSV sickness, who is more at risk, and how serious the illness can be."

Another important thing the CDC does is they watch closely when people need to go to the hospital because of RSV. They have a special network called the RSV Hospitalization Surveillance Network (RSV-NET) that keeps track of how many people need hospital care because of RSV. This way, they can understand how bad the sickness can get and who might need more help.

The CDC doesn't stop there. They're also trying to make a special shield to protect us from RSV. It's like a superpower shield called a vaccine. This shield can help stop us from getting really sick if we ever come across RSV. They're working hard to create a vaccine that can prevent RSV and keep us safe.

In a nutshell, the CDC is like a superhero team. They're not just trying to understand RSV better, but also keeping an eye on how it spreads and making a special shield to protect us from getting really sick. Their work is super important for keeping us all healthy.

The need for further advancements

Even though scientists and doctors have learned a lot about RSV, there's still a lot more to figure out, especially when it comes to stopping this bug from making us sick. There's this big gap between what we know and what we need to know to keep everyone safe from RSV."

Right now, there isn't a perfect way to treat or stop RSV completely. That's a problem because it means some people can still get really sick from it. So, doctors, nurses, and others who take care of us need more information and better ways to help when someone gets sick with RSV."

Another important thing is making sure everyone knows how to stop RSV from spreading. It's not just about doctors and nurses; it's about all of us knowing what to do. That's why we need programs that teach new parents about keeping their babies safe from RSV. And it's not just parents; everyone in the family and even people who are influencers in our community need to know too. That way, they can spread the word about keeping us all healthy.

This teaching about RSV safety can't just be in books or at the doctor's office. We need to learn about it from everywhere, like on TV, social media, or our phones. It's like having messages everywhere we look, reminding us how to stay safe from RSV."

So, even though we've learned a lot about RSV, there's still more to understand and do. We need better ways to help when someone gets sick and, more importantly, ways to stop RSV from making more people sick. It's like we're all working together to learn and share so we can stay healthy.

Importance of RSV awareness and education
RSV is like a big problem, especially for certain groups of people like babies, older folks, and those who might not be feeling well already. This bug is really good at spreading from one person to another, making it easy for many people to get sick. You can catch it when someone who's infected coughs or sneezes, or even by touching things they've touched."

Because RSV can make people really sick, it's super important that everyone knows about it. When we know about RSV, we can do things to keep ourselves and others safe. That's why spreading the word and teaching everyone about RSV is crucial.

Parents and caregivers play a big role in protecting babies from RSV. They need to know simple things like washing hands often to keep away the germs, avoiding being too close to people who are sick, and keeping little ones away from crowded places during the time when RSV is more common."

When we learn about these simple steps, we can help stop RSV from spreading and making more people sick. It's like a shield that we create by learning how to keep the germs away. And when we tell others about it, we're protecting our friends and family too.

Chapter 2

Signs & Symptoms of RSV

Early Indicators of RSV

RSV is a kind of virus that can affect how we breathe. What's interesting is that the way RSV makes us feel can be different for different people. It's like a sneaky virus that acts differently depending on how old we are and if we're already feeling okay or not.

For some of us, RSV might feel like having a cold – you know, a runny nose, maybe a cough, and feeling a bit under the weather. But for others, especially if we're babies or our health isn't so good, RSV can make us feel much worse. It's like having a really hard time breathing, feeling super tired, or having a really bad cough.

So, what happens when we get RSV can be a bit like a surprise – it's not the same for everyone. For younger kids or those who might already be feeling unwell, RSV can be pretty tough and make them feel really poorly. But for some of us who are healthy and a bit older, RSV might not be as bad, and we might just feel like we have a mild cold.

Understanding RSV and how it can affect different people is important. Some of us might just need a bit of rest and feel better in a few days, while others might need more help to feel okay again.

First signs and initial symptoms of RSV in infants and children

In infants and young children, the first signs of RSV infection are usually mild and similar to those of a cold.

These may include:

- Runny or stuffy nose
- Cough
- Mild fever
- Sore throat
- Earache
- Decreased appetite
- Irritability
- Difficulty sleeping
- Wheezing or rapid breathing in severe cases

Symptoms of RSV in infants and young children usually appear within 4 to 6 days after exposure to the virus.

Early warning signs in adults with chronic medical conditions.

In adults with chronic medical conditions, RSV can cause more severe symptoms. Early warning signs of RSV in adults with chronic medical conditions may include:

- Shortness of breath
- Wheezing
- Rapid breathing
- Chest pain or discomfort

- High fever
- Severe cough
- Bluish color of the skin due to lack of oxygen (cyanosis)

If you have a chronic medical condition and experience any of these symptoms, it is important to seek medical attention right away

Differentiating RSV symptoms from common cold or flu
The symptoms of RSV can be similar to those of a common cold or flu. However, there are some differences that can help differentiate RSV from other respiratory illnesses. For example:

- RSV symptoms tend to come on more gradually than flu symptoms, which can appear suddenly.
- RSV symptoms are usually milder than flu symptoms, which can be severe.
- RSV can cause wheezing or rapid breathing in infants and young children, which is less common with the flu.
- RSV can cause shortness of breath, wheezing, and chest pain or discomfort in adults with chronic medical conditions, which is less common with the flu.

If you are experiencing symptoms of RSV or any other respiratory illness, it is important to seek medical attention right away. Your healthcare provider can help determine the cause of your symptoms and recommend appropriate treatment options

Severity and Progression of Symptoms

Description of symptoms as RSV progresses

The symptoms of respiratory syncytial virus (RSV) can vary depending on the age of the person infected and their overall health status.

In infants and young children, the first signs of RSV infection are usually mild and similar to those of a cold. These may include:

Runny or Stuffy Nose: A runny or stuffy nose can be one of the first signs of RSV. It's like when your nose feels drippy or blocked, making it hard to breathe through your nostrils. For babies and kids, this might mean sniffling a lot or having difficulty feeding due to nasal congestion.

Cough: A cough with RSV can start off mild, like a tickle or irritation in the throat, leading to occasional coughing. But as RSV progresses, the cough can become more frequent and severe, causing discomfort and making breathing harder.

Mild Fever: RSV might bring a mild fever, where the body temperature increases a bit. It's like feeling warmer than usual and might make you feel a bit tired or restless. Babies and young kids might feel a little warmer than usual to touch.

Sore Throat: A sore throat with RSV feels uncomfortable and scratchy, like it's difficult to swallow or talk without feeling a bit of pain. It can add to the discomfort caused by the illness.

Earache: Some children with RSV might experience ear pain or discomfort. It's like a dull ache or pressure inside the ears, making them fussier or pulling at their ears.

Decreased Appetite: RSV can cause a loss of interest in eating. Babies might feed less than usual or seem less interested in milk or food, which could lead to reduced intake.

Irritability: Children, especially infants, might feel more irritable or fussy than usual. They might cry more and seem less settled or content.

Difficulty Sleeping: RSV can disrupt sleep patterns, making it hard for babies or young kids to rest peacefully. It might lead to more frequent waking, restlessness, or trouble falling asleep due to discomfort or breathing difficulties.

Wheezing or Rapid Breathing in Severe Cases: As RSV worsens, breathing might become more challenging. Wheezing, a whistling sound while breathing, or rapid breathing, where the chest moves faster than usual, might occur. This can be especially alarming and requires immediate attention, especially in severe cases.

In adults with chronic medical conditions, RSV can cause more severe symptoms. These include:

Shortness of Breath: RSV can make it hard for adults with chronic medical conditions to breathe normally. It feels like there's not enough air, making them feel breathless or as if they can't get enough air into their lungs. They might feel like they need to take deeper or faster breaths.

Wheezing: Wheezing is a whistling or squeaky sound while breathing. It's like a musical sound that comes from the chest while inhaling or exhaling. It can make breathing uncomfortable and might be more pronounced during RSV infections.

Rapid Breathing: With RSV, adults might breathe faster than usual. It's like their chest moving quickly up and down, trying to get more air. This rapid breathing might feel tiring and make them feel breathless.

Chest Pain or Discomfort: RSV can cause chest pain or discomfort. It's like a pressure or heaviness in the chest, sometimes sharp or dull. This discomfort can be due to the strain on the lungs or difficulty in breathing properly.

High Fever: RSV might cause a high fever in adults with chronic medical conditions. This is when the body temperature increases significantly above the normal range, leading to feelings of shivering, sweating, and overall weakness.

Severe Cough: A severe cough with RSV in adults can be persistent and intense. It's like coughing very hard and often, causing discomfort and sometimes leading to chest soreness.

Bluish Color of the Skin (Cyanosis): Cyanosis occurs when the skin, lips, or nails turn bluish due to a lack of oxygen in the blood. It's like a bluish or purplish tint, indicating that the body isn't getting enough oxygen. This is a severe sign and requires immediate medical attention.

Recognizing these warning signs is crucial in adults with chronic medical conditions as RSV can worsen their existing health issues and lead to severe complications. Seeking prompt medical care is essential to manage these symptoms effectively and prevent the progression of the illness.

Identifying severe symptoms that require immediate medical attention

RSV can be particularly dangerous for vulnerable populations, including premature and very young infants, children with chronic lung disease or congenital heart disease, and people who are over age 65 4. In severe cases, RSV can lead to pneumonia and bronchiolitis, which can cause additional symptoms such as:

- Difficult, short, or fast breathing
- Wheezing
- Bluish skin due to lack of oxygen (cyanosis)
- High fever
- Severe cough

The symptoms of RSV can vary depending on the age of the person infected. If you have a chronic medical condition and experience any of these symptoms, it is important to seek medical attention right away.

According to a study by King's College London, the symptoms of early COVID-19 infection differ among age groups and between men and women. These differences are most notable between younger age groups (16 to 59 years) compared to older age groups (60 to 80 years and over), and men have different symptoms compared to women in the early stages of COVID-19 infection.

Chapter 3

Transmission and Contagious Nature

Modes of RSV Transmission

Respiratory syncytial virus (RSV) is highly contagious and can spread easily from person to person. RSV can spread through:

- Infected droplets in the air when an infected person coughs or sneezes.
- Direct contact with an infected person, such as kissing or hugging.
- Touching a surface contaminated with the virus and then touching your mouth, nose, or eyes.

People infected with RSV are usually contagious for 3 to 8 days and may become contagious a day or two before they start showing signs of illness. However, some infants and people with weakened immune systems can continue to spread the virus even after they stop showing symptoms, for as long as 4 weeks.

Children are often exposed to and infected with RSV outside the home, such as in school or childcare centers. They can then transmit the virus to other members of the family. RSV can survive for many hours on hard surfaces such as tables and crib rails. It typically lives on soft surfaces such as tissues and hands for shorter amounts of time 1.

Factors contributing to the contagious nature of RSV

Several factors contribute to the contagious nature of RSV, including:

- The virus is highly contagious and can spread easily from person to person.
- Infants and young children are more susceptible to RSV infection because their immune systems are not fully developed.
- People with weakened immune systems are more susceptible to RSV infection.
- RSV can survive for many hours on hard surfaces such as tables and crib rails, making it easy to spread

Preventive measures to reduce transmission

Preventive measures can help reduce the spread of RSV. Here are some tips to help prevent the spread of RSV:

- Wash your hands frequently with soap and water for at least 20 seconds.
- Avoid close contact with people who are sick.
- Cover your mouth and nose with a tissue when you cough or sneeze, and dispose of the tissue immediately.
- Clean and disinfect frequently touched objects and surfaces, such as toys, doorknobs, and countertops.
- Stay home if you are sick, and avoid close contact with others until you are feeling better.

- Avoid sharing cups, utensils, and other personal items with others.
- Wear a mask if you are sick to prevent the spread of infection

Chapter 4

Diagnosis and Treatment

Diagnostic Procedures for RSV

Respiratory syncytial virus (RSV) is diagnosed based on the findings of a physical exam and the time of year the symptoms occur 1. During the exam, the doctor will listen to the lungs with a stethoscope to check for wheezing or other abnormal sounds. Laboratory and imaging tests aren't usually needed. However, they can help diagnose RSV complications or rule out other conditions that may cause similar symptoms.

Tests that may be used to diagnose RSV include:

Physical Exam: The doctor starts by checking the person's body. They use a stethoscope to listen to the lungs and see if there are any strange sounds while breathing, like wheezing or other unusual noises. It's like when the doctor is listening to the body's 'talk' to understand if everything is alright.

Observing the Time of Year: Sometimes, the time of year can also give clues. RSV often shows up during certain seasons. So, if someone feels sick with symptoms that match RSV during those times, it helps the doctor figure out if it might be RSV.

Tests Used for Diagnosis: The doctor might also do a few tests to be sure it's RSV and not something else causing similar problems.

Blood Tests: They might take a small sample of blood to see if there's anything unusual, like more white cells fighting germs or signs of viruses or bacteria in the body.

Chest X-rays: To get a closer look at the lungs, the doctor might take a picture called an X-ray. It's painless and helps check if there's any inflammation in the lungs.

Swab Test: Sometimes, they use a soft swab to gently collect mucus from inside the mouth or nose. This helps to find signs of the RSV virus.

Pulse Oximetry: This is a tiny, painless device placed on the skin, often on a finger. It checks if there's enough oxygen in the blood. If the levels are too low, it might mean the body isn't getting enough oxygen.

These tests aren't always needed, but they help the doctor be sure it's RSV or see if there's anything else causing the sickness. It's like putting together pieces of a puzzle to find out what's wrong and how to help feel better.

Accuracy and reliability of diagnostic tests.

The accuracy and reliability of diagnostic tests for RSV depend on the type of test used.

Rapid RSV Antigen Tests: These tests are quite common for RSV. They work by checking a sample taken from your nose to see if certain proteins from the RSV virus, called antigens, are there. When your body fights a virus, it creates these proteins. These tests are quick and can give results in about an hour or even less.

Blood Tests and Other Methods: Other tests like blood tests or swabs from the mouth or nose are also used to find signs of the RSV virus. Blood tests can help see if there are more white cells, which fight off germs, or to directly spot viruses, bacteria, or other germs. Chest X-rays are like taking a picture of the lungs to see if there's any inflammation or trouble there. A swab from the mouth or nose helps to directly look for signs of the RSV virus too. Pulse oximetry is a little device that checks if there's enough oxygen in the blood.

No Test is Perfect.

Sometimes, a test might say someone doesn't have RSV when they actually do, or it might show they have it when they don't. That's why doctors don't rely only on one test. They look at everything together, like a big puzzle, to make the right diagnosis.

Looking at the Big Picture

When someone feels sick, doctors use a mix of tests and other checks to understand what's happening. They might do blood tests, urine tests, or even take pictures of the body to get a clear idea. It's like putting all the pieces together to see the full picture.

Remember, no single test tells the whole story. Doctors consider lots of things to figure out if it's RSV or something else making someone feel unwell. It's like being a detective, gathering clues to solve a mystery and help someone feel better.

Importance of early and accurate diagnosis.

Detecting RSV early is like catching a problem before it gets bigger. When we find out quickly that someone has RSV, we can help them and stop the virus from spreading to others. It's like putting a stop sign in front of the virus so it can't go further and make more people sick. The importance are as follows:

Preventing the Spread: When we know someone has RSV early, we can take steps to stop it from spreading to other friends or family members. Imagine RSV as a little troublemaker trying to go around and make others feel sick. But if we know about it early, we can keep it contained and not let it spread to more people.

Getting the Right Treatment: Detecting RSV early helps the doctors give the right treatment. They can start helping the person feel better sooner. Hence, fighting off the virus early before it gets too strong.

Preventing Outbreaks: Imagine RSV as a wildfire. If we can put it out when it's just starting, it won't turn into a big, scary fire that's hard to control. Early diagnosis helps prevent RSV from spreading too much and causing more people to get sick at once.

Importance of Seeking Medical Attention:

If someone feels unwell, it's crucial to get help from a doctor as soon as possible. Early signs of RSV need attention to stop it from getting worse. In a nutshell, early diagnosis of RSV is like catching a sneaky virus before it makes more people sick. It helps us stop the virus in its tracks, get the right help, and prevent it from causing more trouble.

Treatment Options for RSV.

Medications and therapies available for RSV management.

Respiratory syncytial virus (RSV) is a viral infection that usually resolves on its own within a few weeks. Treatment for RSV generally involves supportive care measures to make the patient more comfortable.

In mild cases, treatment may not be necessary, and the patient may recover on their own. However, in severe cases, hospitalization may be required.

Supportive Care Measures

Think of supportive care as giving the body a little extra help to feel better while it's fighting RSV. It's like having some helpful tools to make things more comfortable.

- *Drinking Lots of Fluids*: One way to help is by drinking plenty of fluids, like water or juice. This keeps the body hydrated, like giving it a big drink to help it stay strong.
- *Using a Humidifier or Vaporizer*: "When the air is dry, it can make coughing and congestion worse. So, using a cool-mist humidifier or vaporizer is like adding moisture to the air to make breathing easier."
- *Clearing a Stuffy Nose*: When the nose feels stuffy, saline drops can help. It's like a nose-friendly liquid that helps to clear the nose, making it easier to breathe.
- *Pain Relievers for Comfort*: Sometimes, RSV can make the body feel achy or feverish. Over-the-counter pain relievers like acetaminophen or ibuprofen can help with fever and any discomfort.
- *Plenty of Rest:* Rest is like giving the body time to fight off the virus. It's important to rest a lot, just like taking a break to feel better.

Understanding Antibiotics

RSV is caused by a virus, not bacteria. Antibiotics are like soldiers that fight bacteria, not viruses. So, they don't work for RSV. But if RSV leads to another problem caused by bacteria, then doctors might use antibiotics to treat that issue.

In a nutshell, when RSV isn't too serious, the body can often handle it alone. But if it makes someone feel very sick, doctors have these helpful ways to make things more comfortable while the body fights off the virus.

Effectiveness and limitations of treatments

There is no specific treatment for RSV, and most people recover on their own within a few weeks. Supportive care measures can help relieve symptoms and make the patient more comfortable.

Hospital Care for Severe Cases:

If someone gets really, really sick because of RSV, they might need to go to the hospital. It's like going to a place where doctors have special tools to help when things get tough.

- *Intravenous (IV) fluids*: Sometimes, when the body is very dehydrated, doctors give fluids directly into a vein through a small tube to keep the body hydrated and strong.

- **Oxygen and Breathing Machines**: In some severe cases, when breathing becomes very hard, the hospital might give oxygen or even use a special machine to help with breathing. It's like giving a little extra help to the body to breathe better.

Treatments Not Recommended:

Even though RSV can be tough, there are some things that doctors say won't help. Treatments like bronchodilators, epinephrine, certain types of saline, steroids, and antibiotics don't work for RSV. It's like these treatments are not the right tools to fight this specific virus."

In a nutshell, there isn't a special medicine to directly fight RSV, but hospitals have ways to help when it gets very serious. Knowing what works and what doesn't helps doctors give the best care to help someone feel better.

Supporting the body's natural defenses during RSV infection.

The body's natural defenses play an important role in fighting off respiratory infections such as RSV. Here are some ways to support the body's natural defenses during RSV infection:

Getting Plenty of Rest: Rest is like giving our body a break so it can focus on fighting the virus. It's like when we take a break after playing hard to recharge and feel better.

Drinking Lots of Fluids: Drinking fluids is like giving our body a big drink to stay strong. Water, juice, or soup can help keep us hydrated and help our body fight the virus better.

Eating Healthy Foods: Eating fruits and veggies is like giving our body superpowers. They have vitamins that help our immune system fight off the bad virus. It's like eating colorful foods to make us stronger.

Avoiding Smoking and Smoke Exposure: Smoke is like a cloud that makes it harder for our body to fight the virus. Staying away from smoke is like giving our body a clear path to fight the virus without any extra trouble.

Keeping Clean Hands: Washing our hands is like a superhero move. It stops the virus from spreading to others. It's like a magic trick that keeps us and our friends safe.

Covering Mouth and Nose: When we cough or sneeze into our elbows or tissues, it's like trapping the virus so it can't fly to others. It's a way of being polite to keep everyone safe.

Using a Humidifier and Nose Drops: "When the air is dry or our nose feels stuffy, using a humidifier and nose drops is like giving our nose a little help. It makes it easier to breathe and keeps our nose happy.

Taking Pain Relievers: Sometimes, when the virus makes us feel achy or feverish, taking pain relievers can help us feel better. It's like making ourselves more comfortable while the body fights off the virus.

In a nutshell, doing these things helps our body become stronger and better at fighting the bad virus. It's like giving our body a team of helpers to win the fight against the virus and help us feel better.

Home Care and Management
Comfort measures for infants and young children

Infants and young children with RSV may experience discomfort due to symptoms such as coughing, congestion, and fever. Here are some comfort measures that can help alleviate these symptoms:

- Use a cool-mist humidifier or vaporizer to moisten the air and help ease congestion and coughing.
- Use saline nasal drops and suctioning to clear a stuffy nose.
- Give your child plenty of fluids to prevent dehydration.
- Use over-the-counter pain relievers such as acetaminophen (Tylenol) or ibuprofen (Advil) to reduce fever and relieve pain.
- Dress your child in light clothing to prevent overheating.
- Offer your child plenty of rest and quiet activities to help them recover

Creating a conducive environment for recovery at home

Creating a comfortable and supportive environment at home can help patients with RSV recover more quickly. Here are some tips for creating a conducive environment for recovery at home:

- Keep the home clean and well-ventilated to prevent the spread of germs.
- Use a cool-mist humidifier or vaporizer to moisten the air and help ease congestion and coughing.
- Use saline nasal drops and suctioning to clear a stuffy nose.
- Encourage the patient to drink plenty of fluids to prevent dehydration.
- Offer the patient plenty of rest and quiet activities to help them recover.
- Dress the patient in light clothing to prevent overheating.
- Use over-the-counter pain relievers such as acetaminophen (Tylenol) or ibuprofen (Advil) to reduce fever and relieve pain

Guidelines for monitoring symptoms at home

If you or someone you know is recovering from respiratory syncytial virus (RSV) at home, it is important to monitor symptoms closely. Here are some guidelines for monitoring symptoms at home

- *Checking Oxygen Levels*: Use a small machine called a pulse oximeter. It helps check how much oxygen is in the body. It's like a little helper to see if the body is getting enough air.
- *Watching for Dehydration Signs*: Dehydration is when the body doesn't have enough water. Signs like a dry mouth, less pee, or pee that looks very yellow can show that the body needs more water.
- *Looking for Worsening Symptoms*: Some signs can show that things are getting worse. It's like red flags telling us to get help, such as trouble breathing, chest pain, or lips turning blue.
- *Staying in Touch with the Doctor*: Talking to the doctor and following their advice is like having a wise friend to guide us. They can tell us what to watch out for and when to ask for more help.

In short, keeping an eye on symptoms helps make sure the person getting better from RSV is on the right track. It's like being a caring friend, watching out for any signs that might need a little extra help.

Red flags indicating worsening conditions

RSV can be particularly dangerous for vulnerable populations, including premature and very young infants, children with chronic lung disease or congenital heart disease, and people who are over age 65. In severe cases, RSV can lead to pneumonia and bronchiolitis, which can cause additional symptoms such as:

- Difficult, short, or fast breathing
- Wheezing
- Bluish skin due to lack of oxygen (cyanosis)
- High fever
- Severe cough

If you or someone you know experiences any of these symptoms, it is important to seek medical attention right away.

Steps to take when symptoms worsen

If you or someone you know experiences worsening symptoms of RSV, it is important to seek medical attention right away. Here are some steps to take when symptoms worsen:

- Call your healthcare provider or emergency services immediately.
- Follow their instructions for seeking medical attention.
- If you are experiencing severe symptoms, such as difficulty breathing or chest pain, call emergency services right away.

Chapter 5

RSV and COVID-19

Overlapping symptoms and diagnostic challenges between RSV and COVID-19

RSV and COVID-19 are like two friends who sometimes dress similarly but have their own distinct personalities. They both can make us feel unwell in ways that are quite alike, yet there are also some unique features that set them apart.

Shared Symptoms: Think of RSV and COVID-19 as having a common symptoms. They both might result to a fever, a cough, or difficulties breathing. These symptoms make us feel under the weather.

Differentiating Traits: Even though they've their unique traits, COVID-19 has its special traits. It might come along with losing the sense of taste or smell, something that RSV doesn't usually do.

Diagnoses: Diagnosing these illnesses requires professionalism because they both paint a similar picture with symptoms like coughing and breathing troubles, making it challenging to tell them apart.

Spotting Clues: To distinguish between them, doctors search for clues. COVID-19 sometimes introduces stomach problems like nausea or diarrhea, which RSV doesn't often bring.

In essence, while RSV and COVID-19 share common ground in how they make us feel unwell, they also have their unique traits. This duality can sometimes trick healthcare personnel trying to distinguish between the two, but they use specific signs to solve the puzzle.

Impact of the COVID-19 pandemic on RSV transmission and cases

The COVID-19 pandemic has had a significant impact on the transmission of respiratory syncytial virus (RSV). During the peak of the pandemic, public health measures such as social distancing and mask-wearing helped to reduce the spread of RSV. However, as these measures have been relaxed, there has been an increase in RSV cases in some parts of the world.

The correlation between the COVID-19 pandemic and RSV transmission is more complicated than initially thought. The implementation of public health measures such as social distancing and mask-wearing during the COVID-19 pandemic led to a significant reduction in RSV activity. However, as these measures have been relaxed, there has been an increase in RSV cases in some parts of the world.

The impact of the COVID-19 pandemic on RSV transmission has been observed in several countries. For example, in the United States, RSV activity was low during the 2020-2021 season, but there was a sharp increase in RSV cases in the summer of 2021. In Australia, RSV cases were at an all-time low during the winter of 2020, but there was a surge in cases during the summer of 2021.

The increase in RSV cases after the relaxation of public health measures during the COVID-19 pandemic can be attributed to several factors. For example, the reduced exposure to RSV during the pandemic may have led to a decrease in immunity to the virus, making people more susceptible to infection. In addition, the relaxation of public health measures may have led to an increase in social mixing, which can facilitate the spread of RSV.

The COVID-19 pandemic has had a significant impact on the transmission of RSV. Public health measures such as social distancing and mask-wearing have helped to reduce the spread of RSV during the pandemic. However, as these measures have been relaxed, there has been an increase in RSV cases in some parts of the world. It is important to continue monitoring RSV activity and taking appropriate measures to prevent the spread of the virus.

Co-infections and their implications

Co-infections with respiratory syncytial virus (RSV) and COVID-19 are possible, but they're relatively rare. Co-infections can make it more difficult to diagnose and treat these illnesses. In some cases, co-infections can lead to more severe illness and complications.

Co-infections with RSV and COVID-19 can occur in people of all ages, but they're more common in people with weakened immune systems. Co-infections can make it more difficult to diagnose and treat these illnesses because the symptoms of RSV and COVID-19 can be similar. In addition, co-infections can lead to more severe illness and complications, such as pneumonia and acute respiratory distress syndrome (ARDS).

The implications of co-infections with RSV and COVID-19 are not yet fully understood. However, studies have shown that co-infections can lead to more severe illness and complications than infections with either virus alone. In addition, co-infections can make it more difficult to diagnose and treat these illnesses, which can lead to delays in treatment and poorer outcomes for patients.

It is important to seek medical attention if you experience symptoms of RSV or COVID-19. Your healthcare provider can help determine the cause of your symptoms and recommend appropriate treatment. If you're diagnosed with a co-infection, your healthcare provider will work with you to develop a treatment plan that addresses both infections.

Co-infections with RSV and COVID-19 are possible, but they're relatively rare. Co-infections can make it more difficult to diagnose and treat these illnesses and can lead to more severe illness and complications. It is important to seek medical attention if you experience symptoms of RSV or COVID-19, and to follow your healthcare provider's instructions for treatment.

Strategies for healthcare providers in diagnosing and treating RSV amidst COVID-19 concerns

Healthcare providers face unique challenges in diagnosing and treating respiratory syncytial virus (RSV) amidst COVID-19 concerns. The symptoms of RSV and COVID-19 can be similar, which can make it difficult to diagnose these illnesses. In addition, co-infections with RSV and COVID-19 are possible, but they are relatively rare.

To address these challenges, healthcare providers should consider the following strategies:

- Use laboratory testing to confirm the diagnosis of RSV and COVID-19.
- Follow infection control guidelines to prevent the spread of RSV and COVID-19.
- Consider the possibility of co-infections with RSV and COVID-19.
- Monitor patients closely for signs of worsening symptoms and complications.
- Develop treatment plans that address both RSV and COVID-19 infections 2.

Public health measures to address RSV and COVID-19 simultaneously

Public health measures can help address RSV and COVID-19 simultaneously. Here are some strategies that can be used to prevent the spread of RSV and COVID-19:

- Encourage vaccination against COVID-19 and RSV.
- Promote good hygiene practices, such as frequent hand washing and wearing masks.
- Encourage physical distancing and avoiding large gatherings.
- Increase testing and contact tracing to identify and isolate infected individuals.
- Implement infection control measures in healthcare settings to prevent the spread of RSV and COVID-19.

Lessons learned from the pandemic for RSV prevention and control.

The COVID-19 pandemic has highlighted the importance of infection prevention and control measures in preventing the spread of respiratory illnesses such as RSV. Here are some lessons learned from the pandemic for RSV prevention and control:

- Public health measures such as social distancing and mask-wearing can help prevent the spread of RSV.
- Vaccines can be effective in preventing RSV infections.

- Co-infections with RSV and COVID-19 are possible, but they are relatively rare.
- Healthcare providers should consider the possibility of co-infections when diagnosing and treating patients with respiratory illnesses.
- Early diagnosis and treatment of RSV can help prevent complications and improve outcomes 4.

Healthcare providers face unique challenges in diagnosing and treating RSV amidst COVID-19 concerns. To address these challenges, healthcare providers should use laboratory testing to confirm the diagnosis of RSV and COVID-19, follow infection control guidelines, consider the possibility of co-infections, monitor patients closely, and develop treatment plans that address both RSV and COVID-19 infections. Public health measures can help address RSV and COVID-19 simultaneously by encouraging vaccination, promoting good hygiene practices, encouraging physical distancing, increasing testing and contact tracing, and implementing infection control measures. The COVID-19 pandemic has highlighted the importance of infection prevention and control measures in preventing the spread of respiratory illnesses such as RSV.

Chapter 6

Prevention and Immunization
Preventive Measures Against RSV

Respiratory syncytial virus (RSV) is a common respiratory virus that usually causes mild, cold-like symptoms. However, it can be dangerous for babies, toddlers, and older adults. Here are some preventive measures against RSV:

- Wash your hands frequently with soap and water for at least 20 seconds.
- Use hand sanitizer when soap and water are not available.
- Avoid touching your face, especially your mouth, nose, and eyes.
- Cover your mouth and nose with a tissue or your elbow when you cough or sneeze, and dispose of the tissue immediately.
- Clean and disinfect frequently touched objects and surfaces, such as toys, doorknobs, and countertops.
- Use a cool-mist humidifier or vaporizer to moisten the air and help ease congestion and coughing.
- Use saline nasal drops and suctioning to clear a stuffy nose.
- Encourage physical distancing – particularly in shared spaces, such as waiting rooms.

Importance of vaccination, hygiene, and lifestyle choices in preventing RSV

Vaccination, hygiene, and lifestyle choices are important in preventing RSV. Here are some strategies that can be used to prevent RSV:

- *Vaccination:* Vaccines are available to protect infants, toddlers, and adults 60 years and older from severe RSV illness.
- *Hygiene:* Good hygiene practices, such as frequent hand washing and avoiding close contact with people who are sick, can help prevent the spread of RSV 1.
- *Lifestyle choices:* Lifestyle choices such as getting enough sleep, eating a healthy diet, and exercising regularly can help boost the immune system and reduce the risk of RSV.

Strategies for reducing the risk of RSV infection in various settings

Strategies for reducing the risk of RSV infection in various settings include:

- *Healthcare settings:* Healthcare providers should follow infection control guidelines to prevent the spread of RSV. Patients with respiratory symptoms should be isolated, and healthcare providers should wear personal protective equipment.
- Home settings: Good hygiene practices, such as frequent hand washing and avoiding close contact

with people who are sick, can help prevent the spread of RSV in the home.

- *Childcare settings*: Childcare providers should follow infection control guidelines to prevent the spread of RSV. Children with respiratory symptoms should be isolated, and toys and other objects should be cleaned and disinfected frequently.
- *School settings:* Schools should follow infection control guidelines to prevent the spread of RSV. Students with respiratory symptoms should be isolated, and classrooms and other areas should be cleaned and disinfected frequently.

Community-based interventions for RSV prevention

- Community-based interventions can help prevent the spread of RSV. Here are some strategies that can be used to prevent RSV in the community:
- Public education campaigns: Public education campaigns can help raise awareness about RSV and how to prevent its spread.
- Vaccination clinics: Vaccination clinics can help increase vaccination rates and prevent the spread of RSV.
- Environmental interventions: Environmental interventions, such as improving indoor air quality and reducing exposure to environmental pollutants, can help reduce the risk of RSV.

Preventive measures such as vaccination, hygiene, and lifestyle choices are important in preventing RSV. Strategies for reducing the risk of RSV infection in various settings include following infection control guidelines, cleaning and disinfecting frequently touched objects and surfaces, and isolating individuals with respiratory symptoms. Community-based interventions such as public education campaigns, vaccination clinics, and environmental interventions can also help prevent the spread of RSV.

Advances in RSV Immunization

Overview of current RSV immunization options and their efficacy

There are currently two types of RSV vaccines available:

- The RSV immunization for babies and
- The maternal RSV vaccine.

The RSV immunization for babies is given to infants and young children to protect them from severe RSV illness. The maternal RSV vaccine is given to pregnant women to protect their babies from severe RSV illness. Both vaccines have been shown to be safe and effective in clinical trials.

The RSV immunization for babies is given in two doses during the first year of life. The vaccine has been shown to be 80% effective in preventing hospitalizations due to RSV in infants. The maternal RSV vaccine is given to pregnant women during the third trimester of pregnancy. The vaccine has been shown to be 39% effective in preventing RSV infections in infants younger than 6 months of age 3.

Progress and development in new RSV vaccines

Several new RSV vaccines are currently in development. These vaccines include:

Nirsevimab: Nirsevimab is a monoclonal antibody that is given to infants to protect them from severe RSV illness. The vaccine has been shown to be 70% effective in preventing RSV infections in infants 4.

mRNA-1345: mRNA-1345 is a vaccine that is given to adults to protect them from RSV illness. The vaccine is currently in phase 2 clinical trials.

RSV/PIV3 vaccine: The RSV/PIV3 vaccine is a combination vaccine that protects against both RSV and parainfluenza virus type 3 (PIV3). The vaccine is currently in phase 2 clinical trials.

Expectations for the availability and widespread use of new RSV immunizations

Nirsevimab was approved by the US Food and Drug Administration (FDA) in August 2023 for use in infants and some toddlers during the RSV season. The FDA is currently reviewing Pfizer's maternal RSV vaccine to protect infants. The mRNA-1345 vaccine and the RSV/PIV3 vaccine are still in clinical trials and are not yet available for widespread use.

RSV vaccines are an effective way to prevent RSV infections. The RSV immunization for babies and the maternal RSV vaccine are currently available and have been shown to be safe and effective in clinical trials. Several new RSV vaccines are currently in development, including nirsevimab, mRNA-1345, and the RSV/PIV3 vaccine.

Nirsevimab was approved by the FDA in August 2023 for use in infants and some toddlers during the RSV season. The FDA is currently reviewing Pfizer's maternal RSV vaccine to protect infants and is expected to make a decision by the end of August. The mRNA-1345 vaccine and the RSV/PIV3 vaccine are still in clinical trials and are not yet available for widespread use.

Conclusion

In the journey through understanding Respiratory Syncytial Virus (RSV), this comprehensive guide has aimed to illuminate the multifaceted aspects of this viral illness, ranging from its origins and historical context to the latest advancements in preventive measures and vaccines.

Exploring the intricacies of RSV, this book navigated through its impact across vulnerable populations, shedding light on its severity, complications, and the pressing need for increased awareness and education. Detailed discussions on symptoms, diagnostic procedures, and available treatments provided invaluable insights into managing and addressing RSV infections.

Delving into preventive strategies, the book emphasized the critical role of vaccination, hygiene practices, and lifestyle choices in curbing the spread of RSV. It highlighted preventive measures across various settings, underscoring the significance of community-based interventions and the effectiveness of existing vaccines.

Moreover, the book ventured into the realm of advancements, delineating the progress in new RSV vaccines and their anticipated availability, illuminating the hope for enhanced protection against this virus in the near future.

This book serves as a comprehensive repository of knowledge, offering a roadmap for understanding, preventing, and managing Respiratory Syncytial Virus. With continued research, collective efforts, and the utilization of the latest innovations, the fight against RSV continues, aiming towards a future where the burden of this viral illness is significantly reduced, safeguarding the health and well-being of generations to come.